THE SECRET OF HEALTHY LIFE

ENGLISH EDITION

KAPILA SAINI

ISBN 978-1-63940-713-2

Contents

Introduction

Healthy body and long life is the desire of every human being. But by making some small mistakes, we play with our health every day. But if we keep in mind some small things daily, we can improve our lives, then we can keep ourselves and our family healthy. For this neither we need any doctor nor any expert. Just keep in mind your food and living habits. You know that the immunity of Indians is stronger from people in any other Countries. You must have seen during the Corona era that we do not have good medical facilities nor do people have a lot of knowledge. And in Abroad, there are Good medical practices, and people are also aware, but still the death rate was higher in Corona, in countries like America, Italy, China etc. It did not make much difference in India because our Indian tradition is such that we are unknowingly associated with Ayurveda. In Ayurveda, there has been an attempt to treat any disease with the ingredients of our daily kitchen Stuff. The principle of Ayurveda is to prevent the occurrence of any disease more than to cure the diseases. In case of any disease, it has to be eradicated from the root. If we are imagining a healthy life, then we have to know about Ayurveda first. Then about its treatment.

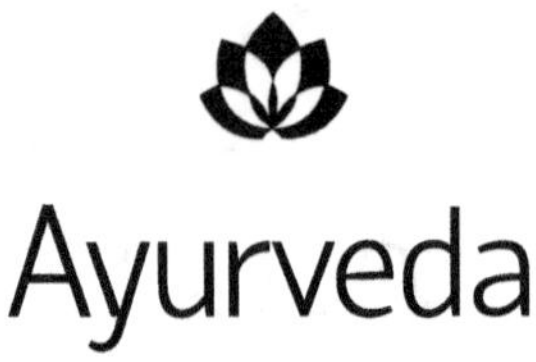

CHAPTER TWO

Ayurveda

Definition of Ayurveda

Ayurveda is a mixture of Ayur + Veda. Which means, age-enhancing science. The name Ayurveda means the nectar of life, in which the entire art of keeping the human body healthy is present. And when there is a disease, it gives a remedy to get rid of the disease.

What is Ayurveda?

Ayurveda is the medical practice of ancient Indian culture. Which means "science of life", in Sanskrit Ayur means "longevity" and Veda means "science." The God of Ayurveda is Lord Dhanvantari. Like other medical methods in Ayurveda, not only the disease is seen, but the cause of the disease along with the disease is also found. Then that disease is treated.

History of Ayurveda

The education of Ayurveda has been inherited from one generation to the next generation in oral form from the lineage of sages. We cannot describe its usefulness in words. Even though the science of Ayurveda is thousands of years old, it is still considered the best science. Today, Ayurveda is also being given great importance in foreign countries. And treatment is being given priority by this. Many such topics are mentioned in Ayurveda in which even today's scientists have not been successful. This proves the antiquity of Ayurveda. The oldest texts of Ayurveda are Charaka Samhita, Sushruta Samhita and Ashtanga Hridaya, written about 5000 years ago. The five elements found in this book space are earth, air, water, fire and sky which together form our body.

Why is Ayurveda the best?

Ayurveda is the result of thousands of years of penance and experience of our sages. Ayurveda is the literature that prevails in the world. After studying it, we can analyze our lifestyle. Ayurveda is not limited only to the treatment of diseases, but it provides complete knowledge of living life.

Purpose of ayurveda

The two main objectives of Ayurveda are to protect the healthy person from disease and second to protect the patient from disease. According to Ayurveda, the basic three elements of the body are vata, pitta, kapha (three metals). If there is balance in them, then no disease can touch you. When their balance deteriorates, only then any disease dominates your body. Today, there are many medical practices, such as allopathy, homeopathy, Ayurveda and Unani. Allopathy and homeopathy treatment provides immediate relief, but it is not certain that the disease will be eradicated from the root. But in Ayurveda, the emphasis is on eliminating a disease from its roots.

Benefits of ayurveda

1. In Ayurveda, attention is also given to the action of the entire body at the time of treatment of any one disease.

2. Ayurveda treatment improves you physically and mentally.

3. The components of Ayurveda medicine are found in herbs, fruits-flowers, vegetables and household things. Thus Ayurveda system of medicine is close to nature.

4. There are some medicines which can be used by healthy people also, it has an effect on the future, disease resistance increases.

5. In practice, there are no visible side effects of these medicines.

6. Ayurveda is such an art of living life, according to this, by adopting lifestyle, you can keep the body disease free.

7. The most important thing is that it is the most affordable and easily available compared to other methods.

8. In Ayurveda, along with the symptoms of the disease, the patient's mind and his physical nature and others are also taken into account.

9. For this reason, there is a difference in medicines for different people even when the disease is one.

10. The most important thing is that chemical substances are not used in this, Ayurveda and yoga together treat incurable diseases, adopt yoga and ayurveda in life and stay healthy.

CHAPTER THREE

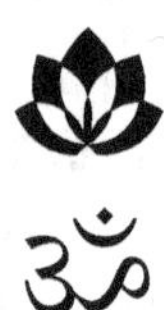

Benefit from the pronunciation of the word ॐ (Om)

Before pronouncing ॐ, we must have complete information about ॐ. You are well acquainted with the word, which is the root of Hindu culture. ॐ is considered a mahamantra in Hinduism. And it is not just one word, but in this one word the entire creation resides. Before the world came into existence, the sound which was echoed in Prakriti Mandal is ॐ. The word ॐ is considered a sign of Hinduism, but it is wrong to associate the word ॐ with any religious culture. The word ॐ is in the world ever since there was no religion but ॐ is in some form or other, the main part of the cultures. ॐ The word symbolizes goodness, strength and devotion. Hindus chant ॐ before all their mantras, Christians and Jews also use the same word "Amen", Muslims call it "Amin", in Buddhist it is called "ॐ Mani Padme Hoon", that Sikh is also "Ik Onkar" i.e. one ॐ.

The word Omni in English which means infinite and never ending. Omni is also actually derived from the word ॐ. That is why we can say that ॐ is not the word of any religion or culture but of the whole creation. Such as air, water, sun etc. belong to everyone rather than to any one. Chanting ॐ provides physical and mental peace to a human being. Continuous chanting of ॐ gives us spiritual and intellectual peace. Through which our soul becomes active and new consciousness and energy are included in the body. ॐ Chanting has a positive effect on the mind and brain. This mantra has such an effect on the body that it is called the seed mantra of all mantras. The sound of the word continues continuously inside and outside our body. Hearing this sound makes one feel empowered.

When pronouncing ॐ:

'A': In the lower part of the body, it vibrates "close to the stomach".

'O': There is a vibration in the central part of the body, which is "close to the chest".

'M': Vibration occurs in the upper part of the body, ie "brain".

The utterance of ॐ gives mental, physical and spiritual benefits. On an FM radio in the US, the morning begins with the pronunciation of the word ॐ.

Importance of ॐ

Monocular Mantras also have special significance in Tantra Yoga. Every word in the Devanagari script has been given a mantra, giving it a reminder. Such as a, b, c, d etc. Similarly, Shrin, Klein, Hriday, Hoon, etc. are counted in Ekakshri Mantra. All Mantras can be pronounced by the combined effect of the air coming out of the teeth and palate teeth, throat and lungs. The sound that comes out of it hits all the chakras of the body and the hormones secreting the glands, by controlling the secretion of these glands, diseases can be shooed away. Today's medical scientists have also claimed that some internal diseases, whose treatment is not available even in medical science. Only regular chanting of ॐ has seen a decrease in them. Especially in stomach, brain and cardiovascular diseases.

ॐ health benefits from pronunciation

1. Digestion: ॐ is not limited to curing mental diseases only. It maintains internal troubles, especially the digestive system.

2. Fatigue: The pronunciation of ॐ acts like a panacea when there is any kind of fatigue. Close your eyes and concentrate your mind by chanting ॐ, which will relieve your fatigue. And by chanting ॐ regularly, body freshens up. And keeps the mind calm.

3. Sleep: If you are struggling with the problem of sleeplessness, this problem goes away within a few days of chanting ॐ as soon as you go to bed. The brain calms down and sleeps well.

4. Thyroid: Chanting ॐ creates vibration in the throat, which has a positive effect on the thyroid gland. It removes the toxic elements of the body. Controls the substances produced due to stress. It balances the flow of heart and blood. If you are nervous or impatient then there is nothing better than the pronunciation of ॐ.

5. Blood circulation: By chanting Om, the flow of blood in the body remains balanced, so you do not have the problem of high and low blood pressure.

6. Intrinsic Health: Vibration in the body is produced by the pronunciation of ॐ, which plays an important role in keeping the internal organs of the body healthy. It also makes the spinal cord strong. And helps the nervous system to function smoothly.

7. Breathing problem: Chanting ॐ daily is beneficial for those who are troubled by respiratory diseases. ॐ pronunciation will make your lungs healthy and strong.

8. Effect on the Nervous System: Chanting of ॐ in the right rhythm and in the right way, that is, when a great vibration is generated in our whole body. This reduces blood pressure and provides comfort to the body. This vibration also has a beneficial effect on our nervous system. This gives the body signals to relax. It also gives mental peace and peace to the brain.

9. Increases concentration: When chanting ॐ with a calm mind 20 to 30 minutes every day has a very good effect on the brain. The vibration generated by this stimulates the memory center of the brain. So that concentration increases for any task and we are able to work with diligence.

CHAPTER FOUR

Increase your Kids Height after 18 years of age

Small height embarrasses everywhere. In schools, colleges, offices and in all places, short height beats you. Not only this, obesity makes people with low height even more disturbing. In such a situation, many people resort to the height enhancing Drinks or Supplements in the market, which cause fatal damage.

Human Growth Hormone (HGH) present in our body helps to increase bones and metabolism. These hormones are very active in children between the age of 12 and 13 years, whose height increases for the next 6 years i.e. children up to 18 years. Height increases. But here we are telling you such ways that children can increase their height even after 18 years.

1. Daily Exercise: Very few people know that our height decreases by a few inches in a day. That is why we feel long while sleeping at night because the body weighs on the spinal code when the body is standing and moving. Which makes the height seem small but if the body poster is kept properly then the change in height will not be seen, for this regular hanging exercise will be required. Which will make the lower back i.e. spinal cord/back bone strong and will not shrink with weight, besides running, jumping and aerobics also prove to be very helpful.

2. Correct nutrition: Fruits, green vegetables, milk and nuts are all good sources of protein and carbs. This improves metabolism and blood circulation in the body. Which boosts growth hormones.

3. Stretching Exercise: The way to increase height is to exercise for 15 minutes a day. This makes the back bone/spinal cord strong by being scratched. This improves the posture and makes the height look longer. Surya Namaskar is also a very good yoga for this. Also, body stretching

is good.

4. Full sleep: Like adults, children also need better and complete sleep. Because even in sleep, the pituitary gland works. That is why it is important to sleep in the right posture, for this position the pillow is not on the head but below the knees, this position will strengthen the back bone as well as stretch it. Apart from this, sleeping in this position also relieves backache.

CHAPTER FIVE

Eat Seeds and Keep away all types of Diseases

We all aspire for a good and healthy life. Do you know that often people throw seeds out of fruits and vegetables in the houses and throw them away? Do not consider these seeds as useless because we can include all kinds of seeds in our diet. You can find many such nutritious ingredients in these seeds. Which can prove to be a better option for your health. Even by including these seeds in your diet, you can cure many diseases of the body. Let's know about some such seeds.

1. Pumpkin seeds: You will be surprised to know that in addition to vitamin B and folic acid in the pumpkin seeds, there is also a chemical that helps to improve our mood. Not only this, pumpkin seeds also benefit a lot in diseases like diabetes. It also proves helpful in balancing the amount of insulin in the body. You can roast these seeds and add them to your diet.

2. Pomegranate Seeds: Antioxidants in pomegranate seeds are best for prevention of cancer and heart disease. Antioxidants that do not allow the blood clot to freeze in the body, plus they are very beneficial for keeping your body in a better shape. You can also consume these seeds to reduce your weight. These seeds can be eaten with green salad. Eating pomegranate is more beneficial than pomegranate juice.

3. Jackfruit Seeds: Yes, jackfruit seeds that you remove and throw on the side can be included in the food when you are hungry. For those who feel less hungry, jackfruit seeds are no less than a boon. Soaking Jackfruit seeds at night and eating in the morning increases hunger.

4. Grape seeds: Vitamin E is found in large amounts in grape seeds. The oil extracted from its seeds is also used as medicine. Grape seeds contain antioxidants, which protect your body's tissues from radicals, thereby

reducing the risk of diabetes.

5. Melon seeds: Melon seeds are considered the best for losing weight. For this, peeling these seeds and consuming it with milk or water, it proves more beneficial.

CHAPTER SIX

How to cure Swelling of Hands and Foot in Winters

Swelling of hands and feet in winter is a painful problem. This problem can occur at any age. In this situation, the suffering person has to face a lot of problems. There is swelling, redness and burning sensation in the feet, especially around the ankles and toes. This swelling problem can occur in any season. But this problem is aggravated in winter, this disease called Chilblance is caused by walking barefoot or sudden change in temperature in winter. Although it is a common disease in winter. But it can be painful if you do not pay attention. But it can be avoided by taking small precautions and simple measures. Prevent cold, wear gloves and socks, sit in the sun and help your feet.

1. In winter, a mixture of candle and mustard oil is very beneficial to avoid swelling and redness of the extremities. Heat the mustard oil in a bowl and then put a candle in it, cook it till the candle melts completely, cool it and apply it on the swollen area and massage with light hands. You will get relief only after applying two to three times.

2. Take some oil in a bowl and heat it on a griddle. Massage the feet with this oil, massage with light hands for a few minutes. This will give blood to the affected veins and the pain will go away and you will get relief, as long as the swelling remains, massage in this way two to three times a day. For this massage, use olive or coconut oil, keep in mind that the room temperature should be normal at the time of massage, do not massage in a cold environment. You can also massage while sitting in the sun in winter.

3. Dough is something that is easily available in every kitchen. The dough is warming. This heat gives quick relief from pain. Make a paste of flour

and wine and apply it on the painful area for 30 minutes, then wash it with lukewarm water. Apply Moisturizer with a light massage.

4. Hot water and rock salt are also effective in Foot Tendonitis. Add rock salt to hot water and keep your feet in it for 10 to 15 minutes. The heat of the water will pull the pain and the rock salt will replenish the magnesium in the body. To protect your feet from dryness, do this procedure only once a day. Then wipe off the wetness. You can add a few drops of fragrant oil to this water.

CHAPTER SEVEN

Why you should not chew Tulsi (Basil) Leaf?

Tulsi is one such plant which along with being venerable, has medicinal properties in plenty. Tulsi plant also reduces air pollution. Due to the many health benefits of Tulsi, people start their day regularly by consuming Tulsi leaves. So that your health can be better. But before consuming Tulsi, we should keep some important things in mind, because incorrectly consumed Tulsi leaves can be harmful rather than beneficial. Mercury is found in basil leaves. That is why it is said that basil leaves should not be chewed. This makes our teeth weak, and spoils them. Tulsi is very beneficial for us, we must consume basil, but whenever we consume it, do not chew its leaves, you can swallow it with water, do not consume basil in large quantities continuously, otherwise it can cause many diseases. Tulsi should never be taken with milk, it has a very bad effect. Tulsi should not be consumed till 1 hour after drinking the same milk.

CHAPTER EIGHT

Benefits of Green Leafy Vegetables

1. Spinach: Spinach occupies a prominent place in green leafy vegetables. It fulfills the deficiency of iron in our body. Spinach is very beneficial especially for women. Women are more deficient in iron, and they need it. Apart from this, it also supplies vitamin A calcium and other nutrients in its body.
2. Fenugreek: Rich in folic acid, magnesium, zinc, copper, carbohydrates, phosphorus, protein, calcium and iron, fenugreek is extremely beneficial for your health. It helps in reducing obesity.
3. Radish: We mostly use radish as a salad, but its leaves are also very nutritious. Its leaves can be cooked and eaten. Which helps protect against cold in winter. Apart from this, it helps in clearing the body pain and stomach problems and blood.
4. Bitter gourd: Bitter gourd is bitter in taste but very beneficial for health. Cleans the blood. Helps in digestion by eliminating stomach related problems. This increases immunity. Protects against diseases.
5. Green Onions: Green onions are found in abundance in the winter season. It increases immunity along with other nutrients. Green onion is beneficial for the eyes and skin as well as the digestive system.

Green leafy vegetables coming in winter helps to keep this system strong in our body throughout the year, so green vegetables should be consumed in winter.

CHAPTER NINE

Cure of Constipation

1. After waking up in the morning, drink lukewarm water mixed with lemon juice and black salt. This will clean the stomach properly and will not cause constipation.
2. Honey is very beneficial for constipation, drink one teaspoon of honey mixed with a glass of water before going to bed at night, constipation problem is eliminated by regular intake.
3. After waking up in the morning on an empty stomach, eating four to five cashews mixed with the same amount of dry grapes ends constipation. Apart from this, constipation is also cured by eating six to seven raisins before going to bed at night.
4. Take the powder of triphala with lukewarm water every day, it will relieve constipation as well as relieve the problem of making gas in the stomach.
5. For constipation, you can drink castor oil mixed with lukewarm milk at bedtime. This clears the stomach and does not cause constipation.
6. Isabgol husk is the panacea for constipation. You can use it with milk or water while sleeping at night. This will completely eliminate the problem of constipation.
7. Guava and papaya are better beneficial for constipation. They can be consumed at any time. Eating them eliminates stomach problems. The skin also becomes beautiful.
8. After keeping the raisins in water for some time, consuming it, the constipation problem is eliminated. Apart from this, after consuming figs in water overnight, constipation problem is eliminated by consuming it.

CHAPTER TEN

Benefits of Jaggery with Warm Milk

1. Consuming hot milk and jaggery daily removes impurities from your body. So that you will not have any disease.
2. If you use sugar along with milk, then you use Jaggery instead, you will keep your weight under control, if you have any digestive problems, then consuming hot milk and jaggery will help you with every stomach related problem. Will get rid of.
3. If a small piece of quality is mixed with ginger and eaten daily, then the joints will be strengthened and the pain will be relieved.
4. By consuming hot milk and jaggery, your skin becomes soft as well as does not cause skin problems.
5. Consuming hot milk and jaggery will also keep your hair healthy.
6. Consuming jaggery with hot milk can relieve you from period pain.

CHAPTER ELEVEN

Benefits of Honey with Milk

Drinking milk is beneficial for health, you know this. But if you add the honey to milk, then you will get many times more benefits. Not only this, you will also get rid of the problems of health, know the benefits of drinking honey mixed with milk:

1. Drinking honey mixed with milk daily is beneficial for your physical and mental health. This helps in increasing both types of capacity.
2. If you have no sleep or lack of sleep, use honey in warm milk at night. It will also improve sleep and make you feel relaxed.
3. To improve digestion, adding honey to milk and drinking is a good solution.
4. This will also solve the problem of constipation.
5. Milk gives you many essential nutrients in addition to protein and calcium and honey helps increase immunity. Both together prove to be a great health.
6. This is a great way to relieve stress. Apart from this, drinking honey mixed with lukewarm milk increases fertility and sperm count.

CHAPTER TWELVE

Eat beetroot daily, the lack of nutrients in the body will be complete

1. Anemia when the problem of menstruation is removed by consuming beetroot.
2. Consumption of beetroot increases the amount of blood in the body, so it is no less than a boon for women.
3. It is very beneficial to eat beetroot in the form of salad or juice. It is rich in iron, potassium, phosphorus, calcium, vitamin D and antioxidants.
4. It has been told in Ayurveda that it not only increases blood, but also removes problems related to urination.
5. Beetroot contains plenty of fiber. Because of which it helps to overcome piles.
6. Consumption of beetroot removes toxins from the body, and due to this the blood becomes clean.
7. If eaten regularly, it increases the immunity of the body.
8. Beetroot increases calcium in the body, which strengthens bones.

CHAPTER THIRTEEN

How to Boost Immunity

Wake up in the Brahma Muhurta in the morning. For a healthy life, one should get up in the morning 2 hours before Sun Rise i.e. in Brahma Muhurta. At this time, due to the air time, the breath, limb and your mind are completely pure. That is why it is important to follow it.

After this, drinking hot water on an empty stomach as soon as you wake up in the morning will purify your digestive organs. Exercise is very important to keep us healthy. Do yoga and pranayam after getting up. This will help you in keeping you healthy and beautiful as well as make you feel energetic.

Take a sun bath for vitamin D. Before 8:00, the sun is very good for your body. Breakfast in the morning is very important for your body. That's why take care of breakfast in the morning and eat nutritious food.

Lunch should be the main meal of the day. Do not drink water immediately after eating the food. Dinner should always be light digestible. Also, stay away from eating too spicy. Be sure to have a good sleep, it is very important for your health. That is why you must have sleep for 6 to 7 hours.

Most people are upset with stomach related problems due to changing lifestyle and not taking care of food. Such as stomachache, flatulence, etc. At the same time, some people complain of not having a well cleaned stomach. In this article, we are telling you some remedies, which you can get rid of the problem of not having a clean stomach.

If you are troubled by indigestion then you should take Peppermint which helps to cleanse the stomach. It can also be used as a sauce. Toast fennel and white cumin powder first on the griddle and then grind it together, consume this powder either once a day or if the stomach is more troubled with the problem of not being clean, then consume it two to three times.